On The Lean:
Lose Weight &
Maintain

By Troy Moore

Table of Content

Introduction

Written by Troy Moore, a Philadelphia bus driver that chose to lose weight after being told by his primary doctor that he was at a high risk for becoming a diabetic. Diabetes runs in my family. My father has it along with three of my father's brothers who have passed away. Seeing how diabetes affects family, friends and co-workers, I have chosen to make a change by losing weight, eating right, exercising, limiting my sugar and carbohydrates and doing what I need to do to not become a diabetic, and so far I am winning.

After going to my doctor and taking an A1C blood test and getting the results, my doctor told me my A1C was borderline of me being pre-diabetic. I was told by my doctor to cut back the sugar and carbohydrates which I almost thought would be impossible for me to do because I loved juice, cakes, pies and chips, but now I have done it and lost about 25 pounds within 8 months and a total of 50 pounds in a year and a half by cutting back on those same foods I loved. I have eaten right and walked daily. I was 240 pounds with very bad eating habits and now I weigh close to 190. I never thought in a million years I would be about 190 pounds. So, If I can do it, so can you. I stayed focused and maintained. I want to show you how I did it and everything I did to make it happen, and hopefully I can help people out there to do the same.

Let me just say this before we go any further: Losing weight is 80% mental. Yes, losing weight is having the desire to live and maintain a healthy lifestyle. That's all it is folks. That's how I dropped the pounds. I changed my mentality and decided to eat healthy, exercise and live a healthier lifestyle. You have to have the desire and motivation to want to lose weight, if not your going to fail. I am going to be straight forward, honest, real and very detailed about everything you need to be doing to drop the pounds. I am not just someone that wrote a book just to be writing it. I lost weight, and diabetes runs in my family which gives me the right to speak on weight loss. I am not a doctor or specialist. My name is Troy Moore and I am a regular person just like you. I work a regular 9 to 5 job like you. I am not a specialist of any kind. I am just a person who chose to lose weight. You can see my photos as proof that hard work does pay off and it did for me and it will for you if you're ready to drop the pounds. Let me begin.

1. Diabetes

Diabetes runs in my family, on my father's side. My mother was just diagnosed with having type 2 diabetes recently. Even though diabetes is hereditary, as many professionals would say, I am a black American male over 40 years old who has a family history of diabetes and have not got diabetes yet. Can it happen still sometime in the future perhaps? I will do my best to take care of myself, eat healthy, maintain a good weight, limit my sugar, starch and carbohydrate intake to keep diabetes away from entering my body as long as I can. I was a truck driver in Philadelphia in the year 2000 when I came home to see my father and saw he was not looking well at all. I rushed him to the hospital. They ran numerous tests and came back with the news: "Your father is a diabetic." I was sad, but also knew of his bad eating habits which probably contributed to him getting diabetes. The sugary candy, mashed potatoes, fried foods and more were all things my father was eating daily.

I knew he had a very bad eating habit and was not going to doctors for check ups. Just like many other people, he hated going to the doctors. Some people just will not go until it's too late or they get bad-off and sick. Me on the other hand, I stay at the doctor getting check ups and blood tests. This is how I found out my A1C blood test was getting high. If I had not been going, who's to say, I would of probably been a diabetic soon. Folks, it's very important to do your doctor visits. I want to stress that, get up, make an appointment and go. Stay with your yearly doctor appointments. Many people could have avoided becoming diabetics if they only would have went to the doctors for check ups like they should have. Truth be told, this is why people get sick; they never go to the doctor and when they do go, it's too late. Next thing you know the doctor might run blood tests and find out there's a million things wrong with you.

Your body is your vehicle, driving through this world we call life. It's your vehicle. You have to maintain it. If you do not get check-ups, what's going to happen? Just like a car, one day it's going to break down and some things you cannot repair. Follow me. Go to the doctor and get checked out every six months or once a year. Stay with it. I go every six months. I go when I don't even need to go just so they can run lab work and I can hear the words: "Everything is fine." It makes me feel good that I have no issues. Now, where I do hate going is the dentist...but that's a whole other book.

In fact, my father had never been to the doctor or hospital in decades before he got sick with diabetes. I am over forty years old, and I cannot recall the last time my father had been in a doctor's office before he got sick. When he was sick and I rushed him to the hospital and he was told he is a diabetic, they also discovered he had high blood pressure. I mean high, high blood pressure. So, therefore, my father getting diabetes may have saved his life also, because if he did not get diabetes and become real sick—who's to say—the high blood pressure he had and never known would have probably killed him sooner or later. Now that he has found out he's a diabetic the only thing we can do now is learn more about diabetes and how he can take care of himself and control his blood sugar count. One thing I will say, I am happy he got diabetes in the year 2000 at the very late age of 68. He pretty much lived his life, and thank god he is still with me today. My mother, she kind of takes care of herself a little more than my father but she loves her sweets, too much sweets, and so I know how she got diabetes which really did not surprise me when I got the news. Eating all them sweets.

I've been to hospitals and seen what diabetes can do to people. Medical bills, tons of medicines to take, testing your blood sugar everyday, kidney problems, amputation, blindness, the list goes on. I decided after my doctor told me that my A1C was borderline for me being high risk for diabetes and I needed to cut back the sugar and carbohydrates. I did not want to go through what others with diabetes are going through and decided to make a change and live a healthier lifestyle. Will diabetes creep up on me one day and still bite me in the butt? Maybe. I'm not going to just let it walk up on me. No sir, you have to catch me, Mr. Diabetes, and I have news for you. I run very fast. As of this day, I am winning the race.

There are certain medical issues people get that you just cannot do anything about. Glaucoma, enlarged prostate, etc. Certain issues people get as they age or it's just runs in the family and you are prone to get it. Now, you have some medical issues out there that if you change your lifestyle you can offset it for a long time or maybe forever and diabetes is one of them. Like I said I am over 40 years old and diabetes runs in my family. I have yet to get diabetes and do not expect to get it any time soon. High blood pressure also runs in my family. I do not have high blood pressure. It's simply because I took better care of myself than other members of my family, by watching what I ate and working out regularly since my early twenties.

What I am trying to get at folks is, if you know diabetes and high blood pressure is in your family history then make a change. Don't just sit there and say: "Well I am going to get it anyway so I am just going to eat what I want and live my life, I can't stop it." So, you're just going to let the rain storm hit you and just sit there soaking wet. Well, I got news for you, I am stepping outside into the rain storm and I have my umbrella up. I am going to do everything in my power as long as I have breath in my body, to keep diabetes and high blood pressure away from me. People, once you have it, you have it. It's not like a cold. When you become a diabetic, here comes all the other medical issues you have to worry about. I do not want to live like that. I am going to do my best to prevent myself from having diabetes. I will walk, exercise, eat right and maintain a healthier lifestyle from now to forever. It's a choice I have made. You have a choice also. Hopefully you will pick the right one, as I did.

I saw a family friend with his toes amputated because of it. I saw people with limbs cut off because of complications of diabetes. I sat in the doctor's office many of times and saw what this disease does to people. Diabetes is a very serious problem in this world. The only way to fix it is to educate people on how not to get it in the first place even if it is in your family history. Living a healthier lifestyle is the key. You know what I have seen many times? People who are borderline diabetics and still have very bad eating habits and will not stop. Once you are diagnosed with diabetes your whole lifestyle has changed for the rest of your entire life on this earth. You really do not know how scary it is having diabetes till you're up in a hospital and see people with it that have serious medical issues. You ever seen a person that had their toes amputated because of diabetes close up? I have. Fact of the matter is I know of a few people who have diabetes and did not listen to the doctors. They went out and ate what they wanted, ignored everything that they were supposed to do and they are paying A VERY HIGH PRICE for it now.

It is very hard to wake some folks up. I know a few people right now that have high blood pressure and still go out and eat foods they know they are not suppose to have. They know it. Do they listen? No. There's an old saying. "A hard head makes for a soft ass." Some people just do not get it or just do not care about their health. I tell people this all the time. I would rather lose weight and not become a diabetic and eat whatever I want sometimes, than become a diabetic and have to watch what I eat all the time. That's my motto. Just think about it. The holidays come around there's nothing like a big plate of baked macaroni and cheese.

You become a diabetic, you will never be able to eat that again. You can but it will be a whole wheat healthy version. We all know, it's not the same tasting as the regular macaroni and cheese. Let's not forget about that large plate of mashed potatoes smothered with gravy and a slice of sweet potato pie, yummy. I said no, I cannot give that up on the holidays. That's why I lost weight. To eat what I want, when I want by living a healthy lifestyle everyday. Now, it's time for you to make a change and let me help you. The reason why I wrote this book is to help you.

2. Limit sugar/carbohydrate intake

First thing I did to lose weight even before walking was limit my sugar and carbohydrate intake. Notice I said limit, not eliminate. Takes time to eliminate if you were sugar addict like me. People say, stop eating sugar and stop eating carbohydrate. It's not an off and on switch in your brain. You cannot just stop. I could not do it. You have to slowly cut back on it daily. I started off slowly by cutting back the daily sugar and carbohydrate intake every day. My problem was juice. I loved it. If juice was a drug I would have overdosed on it a long time ago, trust me. Every day— juice and potato chips. It was also making me bloated and fat. I would go to the market and buy a small chocolate cake and within 3 to 4 days finish the cake all by myself. I am being very truthful here. I am a real person writing this book and I am going to be very real about what I am saying. I think the only way to reach some people is by being very real and straight forward with what you have to say.

No wonder my A1C blood test result was so high. All the sugar I was pouring into my body. My doctor said to me that I should stop drinking sugary drinks. I responded to him by saying, "You know doc, I do not think I can do that, it's gonna be hard. Doctor you're asking me to do something that I know I cannot do." I was so used to drinking juice everyday. Fruit punch, grape juice, berry punch, iced tea, the list goes on. I just loved juice, and guess what folks? I stopped drinking it. You see what I mean now, about it all being mental? I decided to stop drinking sugary drinks. I made that choice. I found out once I stopped drinking it that I was not feeling bloated anymore and my waist line started getting smaller. Drink water as much as you can. Add lemon, make a gallon, add some fruit, you must start drinking water and lots of it, first off. I know, I know what you are going to say. I hate water. I was not a big water drinking fan either, but I decided to make a change. No soda at all folks. I am telling you this right now folks, leave it alone. This is someone who lost close to 50 pounds talking to you. Leave the soda drinks alone guys. Trying to lose weight while still consuming sugary soda is not going to work.

What I started doing was buying diet juices from the supermarket and stop buying regular juice. Supermarkets carry diet juices, less sugar juices, sugar free powder juice mix which I love and now mostly all I use. Sometimes I will mix a half gallon of sugar free fruit punch powder juice mix and top it off with some less sugar apple juice. I love it, better than the normal juices I was drinking everyday. You have to try different ones and see what works for you. I can say yes for a fact that me switching to less sugary drinks and sugar free powder mix drinks and drinking more water really helped me with my weight loss, no doubt about that. Again, leave the soda and sugary drinks alone. I did it, so can you. Remember I was a juice maniac every day. Trust me when I tell you.

Now, let's talk about sweets like cakes, pies, cookies, ice cream, etc. Yes that was me. Going to the bakery on the avenue buying slices of sweet potato pies, cheesecakes, and my favorite— glazed doughnuts. If you want to lose weight, you have to stop. It's hard, I know, it was hard for me too, but it has come to an end! Sorry guys, no more sweets and junk food. It's not the end of the world. I can tell you this right now, once you lose weight and you really know how to maintain it; It's not going to hurt you to once in awhile cheat and get some cake or pie. I still once in awhile go to the bakery and get some cheesecake but it's once in awhile.

I go out to eat at some of the popular restaurants and once in awhile still get a slice of cake or pie, and my weight stays the same. Again, you can cheat sometimes once you achieve your weight loss goal, I do it. What I bought during my weight loss period was mostly sugar free cookies and no sugar added pies & cakes and low fat ice cream, and low fat snacks. I still ate those products in moderation. I was going to lose weight but I still loved my snacks. What I did was just change and ate mostly sugar free products.

I brought sugar free cookies to my job and gave them out to co-workers. The next day, I found out they ate the whole pack.....like really? Just because it's sugar free do not go crazy with it. It's just a better alternative snack to regular cookies and snacks, that is all.

I have sugar free cookies and low fat crackers in my cabinets now as I write this book. Does it taste the same as normal snacks, some do and some do not. Find which ones work for you. The Dollar Store even sells sugar free snacks. I love sugar free oatmeal cookies. If your trying to lose weight, this is one of the changes you have to do. Cut back on your sugar intake. I did it and it worked for me. After awhile you won't be bother by the different taste of it and it not tasting the same as regular cookies, cakes and pies.

Again, even though you switched to sugar free goodies and no sugar added products remember moderation is the key.

Most people think because they're no sugar added, sugar free and low fat products you can eat as much as you want and it won't bother you, it will if you over do it. Let me explain why. Many sugar free or less sugar products are still high in fat. Read the labels.

Some of these products are still high in carbohydrates, remember that. I would eat 4-5 sugar free cookies every other day to satisfy my sweet tooth. I would get a no sugar added slice of cake or pie from the bakery once in awhile. Still be careful. The trick is to limit your sugar intake, pick better options. Sugar was my weight gain problem and as soon as I cut back and picked other options to eat, I saw pound by pound drop off. Potato chips, mashed potatoes, baked macaroni and cheese all was me. I stopped because I knew starchy foods were one of the reasons people get diabetes. I knew it was time to cut back on it. I would buy low fat cheese crackers, popcorn, wheat bread, wheat rolls, low calorie fiber bars; and I love them.

What I am trying to say is if you guys want to lose weight leave the junk food alone and pick better options. I did it, I used to eat junk food (chips, cookies, cakes, pies, ice cream, juice, etc.) I changed and never thought I could. It took awhile but I did it. I still eat potato chips, and mashed potatoes, and maybe have some regular ice cream once in while, but what I am saying is it's not that often. Only once in awhile I may treat myself. Now that I lost weight and I treat myself sometimes it doesn't hurt my weight gain. I mentally trained myself not to eat certain foods and sweet snacks that much and to only treat myself to them once in awhile. Again, you can cheat and treat yourself if you stay focused and maintain. No one said you can never have that slice of pie and cake that you love so much.

Me and my father went out to the buffet
one day. I had two full plates. I get my
money worth at a buffet, believe me.
Remember I already lost close to 50
pounds. This is a method I use. The day
before going out to the buffet I did not
eat much because I knew at the buffet the
next day I was going to pig out and I did.
Mostly ate healthy, I did sneak a few
pieces of fried fish. I had some carrot
cake but scraped off the icing and I had
some bread pudding. I came home at
about 4pm and did not eat anymore for
the rest of the entire day. Stepped on the
scale the next day— my weight
maintained, not a pound over. You see

guys, follow me. Lose the weight first, then you can cheat and treat once in while. I do it all the time and never gain a pound, it's called portion control. It is a trick to everything, even to retaining your weight.

As to what I do eat. I try to only eat wheat bread or wheat rolls. If I go out to eat, yes I may have a roll or two. Wheat is much better for you. I'm from Philly and love a nice chicken cheese steak once in awhile. Sometimes, I get wheat rolls and cook my own chicken steak sandwiches. Wish I could show you photos, maybe that will be my next book. *On The Lean 2*, we will see. Stay away as much as you can from white bread, white rice, pasta, mashed potatoes and foods that are high in carbohydrates. It turns into fat and will make you gain weight. I did not say stop eating carbohydrates. I said limit them. Remember, again lose the weight first, then once in awhile treat yourself. That's how I did it and I have no problems. You have to give up something sometimes to get what you want, remember that, write it down, store it, keep it in your brain. It works. I can go out right now and get a plate of large cheese pasta and probably drink some regular juice (which I would never do) and guarantee you my weight will be the same the next day because I learned not to overdo it, again remember portion control. That's the secret. You do not have to give up the foods you love, just limit them, cut back and choose better options, that's all. You love your potatoes, like many do, just have a smaller portion of it for now on. I have to tell you potatoes will put pounds on you. Why do you think they feed it to seniors in hospitals and nursing facilities, to put weight on them. I see now why I was putting on weight after eating all those potato chips everyday.

Also, before I move on to the next chapter. There is another issue I would like to touch on about sugar free and diet products concerning artificial sweeteners. There is much controversy about artificial sweeteners. Again, I cannot tell you what to do, eat or use. My thoughts on using artificial sweeteners; to each his or her own. I have no problem using them. It never bothered my weight. I do use artificial sweeteners sometimes.

3. Walk/exercise

First off, let me say this. This is what I have a problem with, when people said they need to lose weight. You will not be able to lose weight sitting there day after day after day after day watching television and not doing any kind of exercise. Snack foods and watching television all day long. If I did that, I would probably still be 240 pounds, maybe more by now. You have to start moving folks. You cannot just sit on your butt all day thinking the pounds are going to drop off on their own. It's never going to happen folks. I am telling you this right now. Weight loss involves putting in work. Do some kind of exercise. Walk your dog, walk your neighbor's dog. Walk around the block for 15 minutes. Go to the park and walk around 3 or 4 times a week. Go outside and chase the birds (just kidding). Take your nephews, nieces or grandkids to the park and run around with them a few days out of a week. Buy a treadmill or exercise bike. I bought my sister a exercise bike. She and her husband love it. You are home, playing music, nobody is there to bother you and you can exercise with peace and quiet. I would wake up 5 am when it was going to be steaming hot outside. I would walk for an hour before it really got hot outside.

I put in work, now I am enjoying the benefits of my weight loss. I look back and say to myself, I really worked hard to get these pounds off, and pat myself on the back. Most people look for an easy way to lose weight by taking all kinds of diet pills. I say stop popping pills and starting walking up some hills. Ladies, you want to fit in that skirt, then put in the work. Walking helps with weight loss and also lowers your blood pressure. Get out and do it. Show me one body builder that got buff without lifting weights and I will show you a fish that can get out of water and dance. I walk mostly everyday like it's a ritual. I enjoy walking because I know what it is doing for me. Not only that, I look at walking as keeping certain medical issues away like high blood pressure. I would rather walk 20 minutes a day and not have to take medicine for certain things if I did not walk. To be fair, some people still have to take medicine for high blood pressure even though they walk every day and eat right. I fully understand and I am aware of that.

Now let's get into how my weight really started dropping once I controlled my sugar and carbohydrate intake and decided I need to get out there and do some kind of exercise. I decided to walk every day and the pounds started dropping like a trash can full of flies being sprayed with a pesticide. Not only did my weight start dropping, my blood pressure was a perfect 110/76. Within eight months of limiting my sugar and walking daily, I went from 242 to about 215 pounds. Now, I weigh about 190 pounds.

I used to be a truck driver and after a lay off went from collecting unemployment, laying around the house then driving buses while eating all the foods that are bad for you and not exercising, that's what caused my weight gain. My normal weight when driving trucks and being physical was around 220, I went up to about 242 when my doctor told me about my blood test and A1C issue. I decided to lose the extra pounds and maybe 10 more pounds to really be on track, so along with cutting back sweets and carbohydrates, I knew I had to get active, so I decided to take up walking and It worked. Yes indeed, I started losing more weight.

Before I get into this any further, I see people who walk for exercise but still eat the wrong foods afterwards, that's a no no. I'm going to say this to make it very clear on how I feel about that.

That's like taking a laxative because your constipated and after cleaning your system out you go get a block of cheese and eat it.

I lost weight because when I started walking, I stayed away from the foods that were making me put on the weight in the first place. If you're going to walk, then eat right, it goes hand and hand. Don't walk 5 blocks saying I'm trying to control my blood pressure but after the fourth block you run into a pizza shop and grab a few slices and say: "I just walked so it will burn these extra calories off from the pizza." Hello, what's the point? I see that all the time. It's not going to work. You cannot eat bad and think walking is going to take care of the problem. Why go to a doctor to get medicine for a cold when you're going to keep walking in cold weather with no hat and no jacket on knowing it's wrong, understand me.

First thing I started doing was walking 20 minutes a day. You don't have to walk 20 minutes, do what you can. 10 minutes here, 5 minutes there and 8 minutes there. All I am saying is get it in. I would say at the most you should do about 20 minutes a day. Split it up sometimes. Walk 10 minutes in the morning and 10 minutes a night. Walk 15 minutes on your lunch and 5 minutes after work. Do whatever you can to get that walking in. Sometimes I walk 40 minutes if it's nice out early in the morning. I may walk 20 minutes in the morning, then walk 20 minutes at night. I still do it. If you need to join a gym for motivation then do it. Again buy a treadmill, grab a friend, get some headphones. Do whatever that motivates you to help you stay with it. Walking burns calories and if you do it everyday, watch what you eat and stay away from sugar and carbohydrates what's going to happen? You will see weight loss, I guarantee you, it worked for me. I am proof of that. Everything I am telling you, I did.

At my job, I come in early sometimes

before I start my shift and walk for awhile. I may walk on my lunch break, depending on how the weather is. After my shift is done I walk 30 to 40 minutes. One thing I see many people do, they start walking and after awhile they stop. I lost 50 pounds and to this day, I still walk just like I am still trying to lose 50 pounds. It's called staying focused and maintain. Do not start and stop, then make excuses. You want to lose weight, stay with it as a daily routine just as it's part of your life. There is 24 hours in a day. You know what's funny, when I hear people say, I do not have time to walk. So, you do not have 10-15 minutes a day to give to take care of your body? Seriously? I told you in the beginning of this book I will keep this as real as I can. I am not holding any punches back. You want to lose weight. I am telling you how to.

I watch my sodium intake, I watch my sugar intake every day, I try to eat right, I try not to snack all day long. Breakfast (oatmeal or cereal with fruit) most of the time. My lunch (roast chicken sandwich on wheat bread) or something light and healthy most of the time. My early dinner (bake chicken, grill fish, vegetables) or something that's not weight gaining making me feel sluggish for the rest of the day. You have to find what works for you and what is healthy. I am a chicken and fish person. I love chicken and fish.

That's mostly my diet. Walk and eat right folks, it works. You will be surprised when you start walking and watching what you put in your body how those pounds start dropping. You may not see any changes in your weight. It may take a few weeks just like me, stay focused and don't lose motivation. The weight will start to fall off, it takes time. If you're going to eat whatever you want like fries, cheeseburgers, potatoes, junk foods and drink soda, etc. and think walking is going to fix everything, you're going to be in for a big surprise. Did that, been there. You're just putting the pounds back on you have lost by walking. You're walking to burn and get rid calories. DO NOT PUT THEM

BACK IN YOUR BODY.

Sometimes I do sets of jumping jacks in my house. At one time it was a struggle. I kept doing them until it got easy for me. I started off doing 20 and did a few sets until I got to the point where I can do a 100 and 3 to 4 sets daily. I remember I could not do 10 without getting tired, which shows I was out of shape, but I kept pushing until I could do many without getting tired. I was motivated. I was eager to lose weight. Now, I can do 100 jumping jacks in sets. Same technique I use with push-ups. There's plenty of workout routines you can do without going to a gym. I to this day have never been inside a gym. I take my shoes off, get comfy at home, play some music or turn on the television and start working out, probably for 45 minutes to an hour daily or ever other day.

I have free weights at home. I try do a few sets of curls everyday. I try to find different ways to exercise with my weights and it helps. Walking alone and eating right helped me lose pretty much all of my 50 pounds. I lift weights just to get strong and toned up. It also helps to burn calories also and keep my weight regulated. If you're trying to lose weight, walking will pretty much be the one thing you need to do as long as you follow the rules about eating right and stay with it. Eat right and limit the sugar and carbohydrates. I walked my way into weight loss then after I reached my goal, I started lifting weights just to tone everything up, that's how I did it. Losing weight takes determination folks, it's not easy. I made the change, so can you. I am over 40 years old and dropped the weight, so I know you can. You're not going to lose 30 pounds in weeks. You did not get your high school diploma in 1 year, did you? You did not learn how to drive a car in one day, correct? Losing weight is a process, let no one tell you anything different. If someone tells you, you can lose 20 pounds in several days without exercising you better turn around and run away as fast as you can.

4. Change Your Eating Habits

A trick I will share with you all is eating light throughout the day helped me lose weight. I eat light and I eat healthy. I was no longer piling my plate up two, three, four times a day. I do not eat heavy anymore.

To me cutting back on the sugar and

carbohydrates was hard. Walking daily was really, to me, the easy part. Changing my eating habits was the most difficult part when trying to lose weight. I had been eating the same kind of food all my life. You do not know how hard it was for me to give up on certain foods.

Remember what I said earlier, it's all mental. Losing weight and eating healthy is a mentality you have to instill within yourself to reach your weight loss goal. You have to want to do it. That's why most diets fail, because people do not have the motivation to stick with it and they throw in the towel and go back to their bad eating habits. Diets don't fail. People lose the will to keep them up and stay with it. The motivation has gone. Remember in the movie Rocky 3, when Apollo was training Rocky to fight Mr. T and Rocky just was not motivated anymore? Rocky was not training hard anymore and Apollo said that's it, it's over, what's the hell matter with you. Diets do not fail, people fail to stick with them, I truly believe that to this day, people simply give up. I started walking and changed my diet. How come my diet did not fail? That is because I stayed focus.

I loved fried chicken, fried seafood, junk food, potatoes, hot wings, etc. I would order 30 hot wings, eat half then wait until late night, then finish the other half.

My biggest problem was eating and laying on top of it at night. No wonder I was putting on pounds. Now, before I continue I would like to say, I am not a doctor, specialist, nutritionist, dietitian, food expert, chef, etc. I am a normal guy that works a 9 to 5 normal job who decided to lose weight, did it and wrote this book to help people. I cannot tell you what to eat. I only eat chicken, turkey and seafood. I stopped eating beef and pork over 20 years ago. Everyone has a different appetite and taste buds. Me, for example in the morning, I only eat oatmeal or granola cereal both topped with blueberries. That's pretty much my morning breakfast. Many people hate oatmeal, it's not for everyone. Once in awhile, I may have turkey bacon, eggs, or even sometimes pancakes, but it's very rare.

Pick a healthy breakfast. Find what works for you that's not going to hurt your weight loss program. Example, having pancakes every morning or fried bacon, home fries, cheese eggs, and a cold glass of juice is probably not a good idea when you're trying to drop pounds. I went through several boxes of cereal before I discovered granola cereal and I love it. Does it have sugar? Of course. I don't eat much sweets throughout the day, so granola cereal topped with blueberries is not going to hurt me. Try wheat toast, egg whites, sugar free jam or jelly, almond milk, 2% milk and low sugar cereal, fruits, low sodium bacon or sausages, veggie cheese, low fat butter, less sugar orange juice, less sugar apple, less sugar grape juice—these are just a few examples. There are many diet juices you can find which mostly all markets carry.

There are so many healthier selections and options to choose from when going food shopping. Most people choose not to pick the low fat, low calories, sugar free items because they do not taste the same. You want to lose weight or not? That is the question. That's the problem, people do not want to give up the bad for good.

When I decided to lose weight, I had to change my eating habits and pick healthier selections. Again this takes time it won't happen overnight and as the weight drops off you will be more focus on what to get when food shopping, trust me, I did. You will go food shopping and look at items and say no put this back, can't have this or that. Soon you will be saying to yourself: I can't believe I actually stopped eating this! This is when you will know you're on top of your weight loss game plan. When you can pass by an item you used to eat and will not get it because you know it's not good for you. I walk pass the large bag of chips all the time. As soon as I would go into the market potato chips was the first thing I grabbed. I rarely eat chips now. Mostly I get these low fat baked cheese crackers. They are so good and better than chips.

Lunch or Dinner

Try baked or grilled foods. Stay away from fried, greasy foods. Stay away from starchy, fatty foods like mashed potatoes, pizza, regular pasta and white bread, as I said before. Stop going to the vending machines and buying the junk food. I see that at my job all the time. Lunch meat and processed food are filled with sodium. Try to get low sodium lunch meat, low sodium products and less calorie items. As I said before I mostly eat roasted, baked or grilled chicken and fish. I make sandwiches with wheat bread mostly everyday. If I do get fried chicken now, I remove the skin. I have cut back on eating fried chicken by 97%. I rarely eat fried chicken. I love baked or grilled fish with some vegetables. I try to eat healthy as much as I can. Do I still eat fried fish or fried seafood once in awhile? Absolutely.

There's nothing wrong with treating yourself once in awhile. I lost about 50 pounds, and if I want to have some fried fish with some cole slaw or a small order of fries, I will. I deserve it. I am a very big seafood lover. I love turkey burgers on wheat rolls with veggie cheese. Chicken salad is another favorite of mine with some wheat crackers. Eat more vegetables. I used to go out and buy hot wings. Yes, I am a hot wings person. Now, I love making my own baked hot wings, instead of buying them at the store and it being fried with all that grease like how I used to get them. These are just a few examples on how I eat and I am trying to show everyone the changes I made from eating bad to good. A few more examples are that I love vegetarian baked beans and turkey sausages. Brown rice with vegetables. Most people do not like brown rice. Trust me, I do understand. You have to know how to fix it. Boil your brown rice. Let it sit in the refrigerator for two days, so it can dry out. Take some oil, put it in a frying pan, sauté some peppers, onions, and some cut up chicken breast or whatever kind of meat you like, then add the rice and stir fry it all together. You just made fried brown rice with vegetables and meat. A healthy quick meal.

For all my pizza lovers out there. This is for you. You like pizza, make your own. Markets have whole wheat pizza crust, add some low fat cheese, topped with your favorite meat and there you go. Sometime you have to stop buying certain things and just start making it yourself, it's much better for you. I love pizza too. I eat pizza probably twice a year. It is a food you have to be careful with when trying to lose weight. Youtube has many videos that can show you how to cook healthy. Remember, fast food means a faster, bigger belly. Fast, greasy unhealthy food is why people gain so much weight. Stay away from it if you want to lose the pounds.

Eat more salads. Add meat to them like I do. I sometimes buy a whole roasted chicken already cooked from the store and break it up and put it into a salad. I am not big on salads, that's just me, but when I do make them, they're good. You just have to be creative when making it.

Again, find what works for you. This is something I want to stress. I am just giving you a few ideas on what I eat and cook. I eat fruits. My choices are bananas, mangos and blueberries. Grapes I will buy every now and then.

A question I get all the time is: What should I be eating? I am going to be straight forward on this subject and talk to you as if I was talking to a friend that wants to lose a few pounds.

This is why I cannot read diet recipe books, because most of the stuff they tell you to cook and eat, I don't eat or like. You ever pick up a recipe book and say, I don't have time making this stuff. They tell you to cut this up, chop that up, sauté this, add that then mixed this up. I do not have time for all that, I have to work. If recipes books work for you, then they do. I for one cannot do them, unless it's simple stuff like making a fancy turkey sandwich. Do not get me wrong, I can burn in the kitchen when I have the time to do so, trust me.

What I found out that works for me is to take everything you like to eat and make a healthy version of it. Some people do not eat fish, chicken, beef, or pork. Many people hate seafood, I love it. Again, I cannot tell you what to eat. I cannot say make some shrimp gumbo. Some people do not like seafood. I cannot say try making some steak in the oven, or try some baked pork chops. Like me, many people do not eat red meat or pork. I cannot say to people, another great dish is stuffed turkey, some people might not like turkey. I eat what I eat and you eat what you eat. Whatever it is that you like, make it healthy.

You like pork chops, stop frying them all the time and put them in the oven. You like fish, bake it sometimes. You like burgers, make your own healthy burgers. I myself love turkey burgers with peppers and onions. Some people don't like turkey burgers. I eat turkey bacon sometimes. Some people do not like turkey bacon, but again this is what I like to eat. I cannot say for breakfast try yogurt. I don't like yogurt as many others also. That is what bothers me when you watch these so called weight loss programs and they say for snack time try yogurt. No, you try it, give me my turkey club with extra mayo and my low fat chips, okay. I am not going to say, hey guys at night when you get hungry eat some oatmeal, it fills you up and makes you feel full. Who's really going to do that, not me, especially at night. I am guessing now that many people that are reading this book are probably laughing saying, yes, this person is the real deal. I can relate to him.

Again, take all the foods you love and

make a healthy version of them. That's my way. I love turkey sausages. I do not fry them. I put them in the oven and some peppers and onions topped with cheese, and yummy.

Fried chicken, make oven fried chicken, it's better than regular fried. Ever had oven fried chicken? Try it. It is good. Some people love French fries. Put them in a pan, stick it in the oven— avoid frying them is another way. Get some whole wheat bread, veggie cheese and buy a roasted or grilled chicken already cooked. Make a grilled cheese sandwich with some veggie cheese and just add the chicken on top of the cheese. You now have a chicken & cheese grilled sandwich, put some tomatoes in there if you like tomatoes. I make that all the time. It's healthy, light and good.

Use wheat pasta, if you like to make pasta dishes. This is what I do when making macaroni and cheese. Wheat pasta, low fat cheese, 2% milk and it's good. I love baked turkey chops with vegetables. I'm not going to fast food places eating that crap. I have not been to a fast food place in over a decade, probably longer, I do not eat that kind of food. Another dish I love to make is turkey meat balls with whole wheat spaghetti. Just because you're trying to lose weight and have to give up a few food here and there to control your weight does not mean you cannot have what you love to eat. Again, just make a healthier version on it, simply put. Example, you love hotdogs. Get whole wheat hot dog rolls. Get the less fat pack of hot dogs. You can go to the appliance store or shop online and purchase a small portable grill to start grilling your foods.

If I am hungry and don't have time to cook, I may go somewhere and get a sandwich on whole wheat bread, or swing by a favorite restaurant and there are many in Philadelphia. I am sure in your area there are many places to get healthy take out foods. I will get a healthy platter, like baked fish or baked chicken with some vegetables or a salad. This is what I do when I don't have time to cook or maybe just do not feeling like cooking. Again, stay away from those fast food places. They will not help you with your weight loss. I see many fast food places popping up now that are all about healthy meals. Some places are very nice and serve good healthy foods.

Cooking your own is going to benefit you way more than going out to some of these restaurants who fry the food in grease and add all that salt to it. There's nothing wrong with going out to eat sometimes and enjoying yourself, just watch it if you're really trying to lose weight. Have you seen some of the sodium content in some of the dishes you order at some of these restaurants, it's insane.

When I go out to dinner at different restaurants, I cheat sometimes, I love me some fried onion rings once in awhile. I am a real person writing this book from Philadelphia, so I am not going to jive people with a bunch of nonsense. If I go out to a restaurant, I'm going to eat and I'm going to enjoy myself. Here's the thing, remember portion control. I won't eat it all. I will pick a healthy appetizer with salad. For the main course I eat half and take the other half home and save it for the next day. As long as you don't overdo it, and limit yourself for the rest of day on eating and watching your calories, your weight should still be good and everything will be fine. I do this all the time. I will not each much of the day before I'm going out to a restaurant. The day after going out to eat, I will eat very light and my weight never changes. What you're doing is balancing everything out. It works for me. My weight still stays off and it stays maintained.

Another trick you can use. If you know you're going out with family friends to eat and you know you're going to have a big meal, afterwards walk it off or exercise a little harder the next few days, that also works for me. This is something I do all the time. Eat what you want and work it all off.

Pick a stop eating time (6 pm or 7 pm). Folks this is a very important thing to do. This is not recommended if you're already a diabetic. If you suffer from low blood pressure or from hypoglycemia this method is not for you. This is something I do. Your body naturally burns calories. If you stop eating at 6 pm, which is my stop eating time, you will notice at night you won't feel tired, sleepy or lazy because you're not still stuffing your face all night long, and what calories you did eat in the morning and afternoon will probably be all burnt up by midnight, especially if you walk everyday. I stopped eating late in the evening and notice a big difference on how I feel late at night. I am a bus driver, so I have to really watch what I eat because I am sitting all day. Again, I'm not advising anyone to do this. Stopping eating at a certain time in the evening works for me. This is a trick I use to keep my weight down. I used to eat all night long and after midnight at one time.

If you find yourself getting hungry at night then have a small low fat or low calorie snack. Keep them in your room. Many times at night if I get hungry I eat a few sugar free cookies. Drink some sugar free or less sugar juice to get you through the night. That is what I usually do. I still come home after work at night hungry sometimes and I will grab a few crackers or low sodium popcorn. I may eat some cereal sometimes late at night. Sometimes I cheat. If I'm really hungry late at night, I may eat a sandwich or some chicken salad with crackers. You will not be able to stop eating without getting hungry later sometimes, we are human. That takes a while to master, and it's a trick that will help on your weight loss journey.

5. Stay Focused and Maintain

Losing weight is easy, keeping it off is the hard part. It's so easy to fall off and put weight back on. It's much easier than you think. You ever see a champion boxer on top of the world, then some new kid comes along and the champion boxer thinks he does not have to train hard for this new kid. The champ gets knocked out. He was not focused and he did not maintain what he had to keep the belt. Same thing goes for when you lose weight and want to keep it off. You have to learn how to maintain it. This is how you keep your weight down.

One thing I will tell you now, is to go out and buy a weight scale. This is mandatory. Know where your weight is. This is how I was able to manage my weight and know if I can eat heavy the next day or if I need to take it easy. Without a scale the pounds can creep back up on you just like that. Go out and buy yourself a nice scale. Check your weight every day or every other day. I check mine every day. I stay on top of it.

One reason people put back on the weight is they have no scale, so how would you know if you're gaining pounds if you cannot check it. You go to the doctor and he says you gained 10 pounds. If you had a scale you would of know you were gaining weight, correct? How would you know if your car needs oil if you're never checking it. Next thing you know your car engine burned out. You're saying to yourself, what happened? What happened was you were not staying on top of things. This is a must and very important that you go out and buy a scale. They only cost about $15.

You can lose 20 pounds and get relaxed,

start eating what you want and just like that those 20 pounds are right back on.

Three letters to remember: D.G.C. Don't get comfortable. That's why people put back on the pounds. Because they lost a few pounds and think that it's alright to eat what they want. After a while and every day they slowly go back to their bad habits and before you know it, they are overweight again. That's why diets fail. The diet did not fail, the person did. See, you could have kept the weight off. You thought because you shedded a few pounds eating certain foods you would not do any harm. You kept eating them every day and after a while your weight is right back on you again.

Perfect example is someone at my job made a carrot cake. I love carrot cake. They offered me some. I said no thanks. I was focused on losing weight and knew if I took some of that cake I would be breaking everything I was working for. While everyone was sitting around eating the cake, I was out walking. People on my job were asking me how I lost so much weight. Are you serious? Carrot cake is my favorite. I did not take one piece of it.

Temptation will come after you every day on your diet. Only the strong survive. Wait until you start your diet. All of a sudden when you go to the market, they have the "buy one box of ice cream and get one free" and it's your favorite flavor, of course. Again, temptation coming after you. If you go over to a family or friend's house on a holiday, birthday, or just visiting and they're in there cooking foods you know you should stay away from. Say no thanks, I am trying to lose weight. I do it all the time. What's going to happen is your going to slip up and fall off. You're going to say I will just have a little. Next thing you know you got more on your plate and you just broke your diet with a plate of fried chicken, macaroni cheese and three rolls. Now, your eating a slice of sweet potato pie. The next day you're going back over there for another plate. As, I said before, losing weight is mental, stay focused on your goal. I am just keeping it real here. I have seen people diet then fall off, what happened?

I see people all the time saying they are trying to lose weight but have a large bag of chips and soda in their hand. People sitting there with a double cheeseburger, fries and cake, saying I need to lose some weight, seriously, this is a joke, right.....your kidding me right? I'm not knocking anyone for what they eat. I understand it's hard sometimes but when I was losing weight, I did none of those things. Did I miss certain foods I enjoyed? Of course. One of my favorite dishes is a chicken cheese Stromboli. I haven't had one since I lost the weight.

It's called will power.

The realest show I ever watched on television was *The Biggest Loser*. That show is real. They make them work out, watch what they eat, limit what they eat and change they whole mentality. Watch the reruns of that show and learn, folks. Remember what I said a few times in this book. Losing weight is mental. You have to say, I am going to lose 30 pounds within the next 8 months and nothing is going to stop me or get in my way. That was my mentality, and I lost close to 50 pounds.

Another reason why people fail in their weight loss journey. A few examples:

They start walking and eating right for 6 days, then stop. Some people just get lazy. This little piece of candy bar will not hurt me. The same thing the next day.

I was on my diet and my aunt made some chocolate cake. I will go back on my diet next month. I'm tired of eating healthy, I miss certain foods I cannot have. I will diet next year.

I'm trying to lose weight, it's hard, I do not feel like walking, working out and eating right all the time.

How do you think I lost my weight? I walked and ate right. When you start talking like that and many do and will even after reading this book, you already threw in the towel, trust me. You want to lose weight.........STICK WITH IT. I do not care if the bakery is giving free cupcakes away every Saturday morning. You take your 20 minute walk, walk past that bakery, look, smile, smell and keep it moving. I do not care if your neighbor is having a beer and all you can eat hot wings and pizza party, say no thanks. STAY FOCUSED. Who am I kidding, as much as I love hot wings I would probably go and grab a few (Laughing). It's free too. Hey, I am on a diet. I am not crazy. Okay, lets move on.

I lost about 50 pounds and I live my life every day as if I am still trying to lose weight. I watch what I eat, I still walk and exercise, I still play by the rules I instilled in myself while losing weight. Eat right, eat less and exercise. Don't get comfortable (D.G.C.). Remember those three letters. I still get out and walk 30-40 minutes daily. I don't eat after a certain time. I stayed focused. I maintained my weight. I beat having diabetes, my blood pressure is great and you can do the same if you want to lose weight and change your lifestyle by eating healthier. It's not an easy road. It took me about 7 to 8 months to drop about 25 pounds and one a year and half to lose the rest altogether.

Everything I just shared with you and told you in this book is exactly how I lost weight, everything. How I ate, walked, stayed away from sugars and certain foods. I started cooking my own meals. I selected healthier options when I went out to eat. I stayed focused and motivated. You cannot tell me you cannot do it. I did it. My A1C numbers came down and are getting better. My doctor saw my weight loss and said I should write a book. Next time I see him on my next visit I will tell him, thanks Doc, I just did. I hope it helps people with their battle in weight loss.

Again folks stay away from the sugars and carbohydrates, walk & exercise, eat right, stop eating late at night and laying on top of it. Stay focused and maintain all you have to do and you will win the weight loss battle. If I can help one person lose weight by reading this book, then I truly accomplished what I wanted to do by writing it!

6. The Aftermath Of Weight Loss

I once was overweight, now I am lean. How do I feel now? Like Tony the Tiger said, "I feel GREAT!"

When I was overweight I felt tired many times. I would get out of breath fast. I struggled sometime just to do every day, normal things. It's very true what they say. Once you lose weight you do have a boost in energy. I am no longer sluggish and feeling tired all the time. I can actually walk for a long time without getting exhausted and winded. Heart disease and diabetes are all things that are accompanied by a person being overweight. When losing weight and exercising and eating healthy, you lower your chances of getting heart disease and diabetes. This is what I wanted to do. I have accomplished it.

Losing lots of weight may alter your taste buds. I do notice it when I eat certain foods. Some food may seem saltier or sweeter. I did not notice it when I was overweight. Maybe because

I was so used to eating those kinds of foods all the time. Some fast food fried chicken places now, I can really taste the salt in the food. I cannot eat those foods anymore. It's just too salty.

Did and do people notice my weight loss? Yes.

Did losing weight improve my sleep at night? Yes.

Did losing weight improve my self esteem? Yes.

Does weight loss really improve your sex life, as many say? Yes, Yes and Yes.

Losing weight and becoming lighter also makes me faster. I notice I can move very fast now when doing certain things. At one time I was on high cholesterol medicine. I lost lots of weight, and ever since then my cholesterol has been great. I am sure eating right and exercising also played a big roll also. It feels great to know I do not have to take cholesterol medication anymore as long as I do the right thing and maintain a healthy lifestyle.

This is why it is so important to eat right. I tell many young folks this. When I was young and their age, I used to eat all the junk foods that they are eating now. Wait till you get older then try to eat those same foods and see what happens. Your body changes as you get older. It's important to remember as you get older, you cannot eat like you use to when you were younger. When I was in my early twenties, I use to eat cheeseburgers and all kinds of greasy foods. Let me do it now, at my age. I will probably be in the hospital so fast. So, as you get older folks, you really have to adjust your eating habits. This is why when people get older they come down with all these medical conditions. All those years of consuming bad foods have caught up to us.

Awhile back I was listening to the radio. They were having a health fair. Free screening and all kinds of free tests for people. I walked in and looked around and the place was almost empty. I said, wow. They are giving people free health screening for blood pressure, eyes, and so on and no one even shows up. It was sad. People were there but It should have been way more than what I saw. It was all on the radio being promoted. People knew about it. It is what it is. People do not care about their own health: there is nothing anyone can do about it.

I said this earlier in my book. I believe if people would just go to the doctors and get check ups, they would find out they are borderline high blood pressure and diabetes. This is the only way you're going to find out. Again, I know people to this day that do not listen to their doctors. They take medicine for high blood pressure and keep on eating foods they are not suppose to have. Honestly, I do not say anything. I just look at them and shake my head because they know what they are doing is wrong. Some people you can talk to, but they have to wake up on their own.

My doctor told me my A1C was borderline. What if I ignored him and kept drinking sugary drinks and eating sweets. I'd be a diabetic right now. I made a change and reversed it. The point I am trying to make is that you have a choice. You are in control. Change your lifestyle and live healthier. You have kids, grandkids, and parents to take care of. They need you, so make a change and take care of yourself.

I am 50 pounds lighter and it feels good. If someone was to tell me when I was 240 pounds, one day, Troy, you're going to be close to 190 and you're going to write a book to help people, I would of probably laughed at them like, yeah okay. Last time I weighed around 190 I was in high school when Run DMC, Beastie Boys and LL Cool J were the hottest rappers out. You know how long ago that was? That was a very long long time ago folks. I am over 40 years old and weighing 190 now from 240. I did it, I did it, I did it. Now it's time for me to take you back to school and show you how it's done. It's your turn.

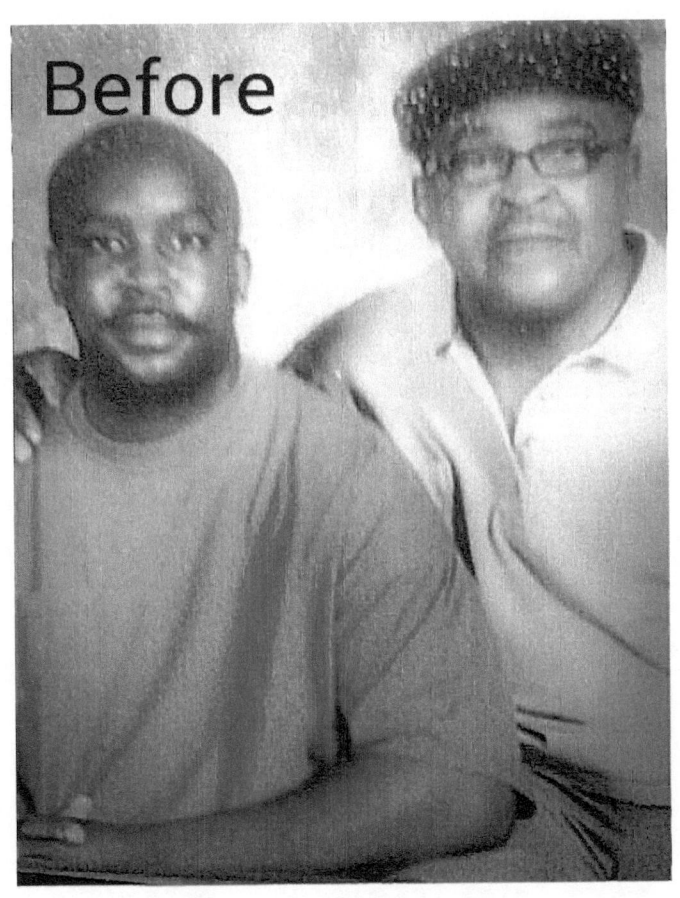

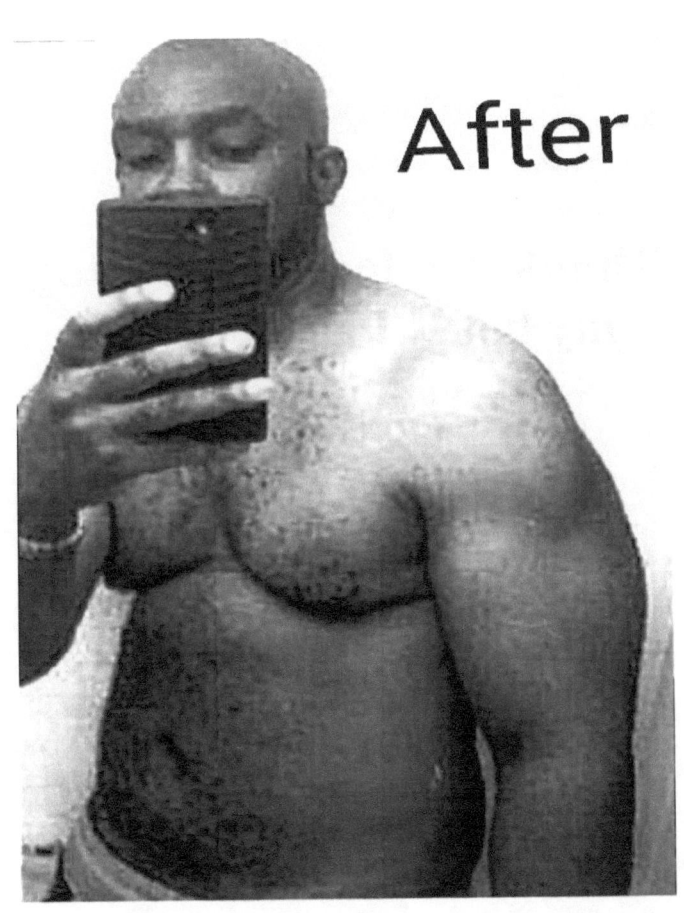

After

Thank you for downloading my book. I appreciate it very much

I would appreciate it if you would leave your honest review of this book. If you have any problems, issues or concerns with downloading this book, or if you have any questions or need any advice on losing weight, you can email me at tmoore780@yahoo.com. I will do my best to try assist you. Thanks.

Thanks & best wishes to you all on your present and future weight loss goals. Troy Moore

HEALTHY CREATIVE CHICKEN & TURKEY
SANDWICHES

Coming Soon

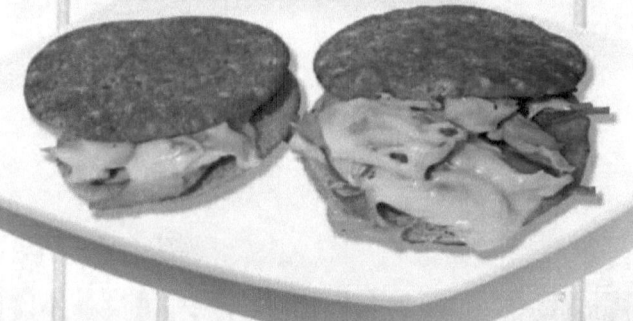

ON THE LEAN 2
SANDWICHES
ON WHEAT

TROY MOORE

Table of Contents